Baby & Toddler
Vegan Feeding Guide

Julia Feliz Brueck

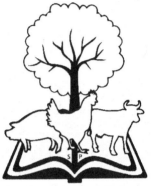

Sanctuary Publishers

ISBN-10: 0-9989946-0-X
ISBN-13: 978-0-9989946-0-4

Illustrations by Julia Feliz Brueck, www.juliafeliz.com

Sanctuary Publishers, www.sanctuarypublishers.com

-A Book Publisher That Gives Back-

Every book sold supports marginalized communities.

DEDICATION

To my children for inspiring me every day to continue my journey of passion towards world justice.

To all parents trying to raise strong, passionate, and aware children. You are not alone.

To Heidi, ask and you shall receive.

CONTENTS

PREFACE

In a world that does not yet fully understand the vegan lifestyle and plant-based diets, I have created this guide to support pregnant mothers, new parents curious about what to feed their babies at 6 months, and those considering transitioning their families towards a vegan lifestyle.

I find myself the only vegan parent in most circles I am part of – if not the only vegan apart from my husband and sons. As my boys grow, I've often wished I could converse openly with other vegan parents about raising our children with vegan values and about what new plant foods they were currently enjoying. For those in a similar situation, I hope this guide will be a way to find reassurance that you are on the right track... even if your playdates do not include any vegan moms or dads.

As a scientist, I want to pass on what I have learned about research and staying skeptical on a world wide web permeated with "fake news" and dangerous pseudoscience. Because of this, it was important for me to ensure this guide and the content I researched and cited was current and nutritionally safe. I was fortunate enough to have the guidance of Ginny Messina on the nutrition sections of this guide so you can be assured it is accurate, evidence-based, and reviewed by a nutritional expert. Ginny is an evidence-based vegan MPH, Registered Dietician with decades of experience in nutrition. She has lent her expertise to guide vegans to live healthily under The Vegan RD website.

Thank you for supporting this guide and for sharing it with parents that may need a little guidance or a nod to let them know they are doing just fine.

ACKNOWLEDGEMENTS

I would like to thank everyone that helped make this book a reality, and especially, Ginny Messina for donating her time and guidance.

1

INTRODUCTION

Following our values

One of the best and most important decisions I have made is choosing to raise both my sons with vegan values. As a vegan of almost a decade, I want to pass on the same values that have made me question my everyday life choices and choose to make my impact on other living beings as small as possible. Apart from helping them develop a connection to other living beings, the most natural way to help them start their own vegan journey is through what they eat.

It feels good to know my sons can reap the many benefits of a healthy vegan diet and at the same time, grow up to know that their food choices are the kindest to humans and non-humans alike. I truly believe this is the best start a child can get - one filled with awareness of where their food comes from because they have the knowledge of why we choose to eat plant-based foods. Raising them with this knowledge will aid in their ability to maintain and nurture the compassion that every child is born with.

Raising strong, healthy, and compassionate children is one of the most important legacies we can leave behind as vegan parents.

Keep It Simple!

Despite being a decade long vegan without health issues and undergoing a healthy vegan pregnancy, hours after the birth of my first son, we were bullied by the on-call pediatrician when she discovered we were vegans. She claimed that vegetarians and vegans could not possibly live healthy lives, nor could children be healthily raised vegan. At one point, she made reference to that one news story most people not well versed about plant-based diets or vegan lifestyles always seem to use against us – the story of parents that starved their newborn by only feeding it soy milk. I realized this story was most likely the extent of her knowledge of veganism. From then on, I felt a need to ensure that other vegan parents had access to evidence-based information for themselves and to share with medical professionals should they need it. While the medical community has a responsibility to evolve with changing customs and lifestyles, we, as parents, also have a responsibility to ensure we are using evidence-based guidelines to raise healthy children.

I'm not anti-doctor by any means. I did not have

any problems during the birth of my second son. We also appreciate our current pediatrician, and before we moved, had a fantastic pediatrician that really knew her field. I've never had any issues with health professionals before this particular doctor; therefore, what I am against is ignorance based on preconceived ideas instead of evidence-based medicine. Unfortunately, this ignorance, which still follows our movement despite support from dietetic associations across the globe, has been promoted and fed by the media. Every once in while it rears its ugly head because of a case of malnourishment or an ill-written article by an untrained author.

My own experience made me want to work against the ignorance I encountered while at the same time support other vegan parents that might need some simple meal inspiration. This is why this guide now exists.

Honestly, feeding my son has not been challenging at all, as some media would have their readers or viewers believe. I don't really use any "superfoods" nor do I spend tons of money making gourmet foods. I do not spend hours in the kitchen, either. As a mom living away from family and friends, saving time is a high priority, especially with a new baby and a very energetic 2.5-year-old. My motto really is "keep it simple".

I hope you will find this food guide helpful,

affordable, and time-saving. Wherever possible, I will quote directly from scientific, medical, and dietetic sources so you can be sure this guide is evidence based.

A Side Note

What happened to the doctor? With the help of the International Vegan Rights Alliance, vegan parent rights are protected at the hospital where I gave birth. They passed a directive based on my case, which requires doctors to work with vegan parents and their rights to make decisions for their own children instead of using their power over them and their ethics.

Should you ever find yourself in a similar situation, you can find legal representatives all over the world through their website http://www.theivra.com/

2

SUPPORT FROM DIETETIC ASSOCIATIONS

I'm not alone in having fears creep up once in a while when dealing with someone who claims my vegan diet is responsible for every tiny little thing that may come up with my health. Although we know we have chosen the best possible way to feed our family in the most ethical manner, one of the most common fears I have read in vegan parenting groups shows through in the need for many to receive confirmation they are doing well in feeding their vegan children.

As you all know by now, the Academy of Nutrition and Dietetics (AND), previously known as the American Dietetic Association, came out in 2009 with a statement in support of vegan diets at all stages of life. Did you also know that the Australian, Canadian, and British dietetic associations have done the same? With more and more support, we, as parents, can feel empowered in knowing that well-planned diets are healthy and safe for our children.

The official statement of the AND (ADA), released

initially in 2009, included vegan under the definition of vegetarian and stated, "It is the position of the American Dietetic Association that appropriately planned vegetarian diets, including total vegetarian or vegan diets, are healthful, nutritionally adequate, and may provide health benefits in the prevention and treatment of certain diseases. Well-planned vegetarian diets are appropriate for individuals during all stages of the life cycle, including pregnancy, lactation, infancy, childhood, and adolescence, and for athletes." Based on several research studies done on vegetarian children, the statement goes on to state, "vegetarian children and adolescents have lower intakes of cholesterol, saturated fat, and total fat, and higher intakes of fruits, vegetables, and fiber than non-vegetarians", as well as tend to be "leaner and to have lower serum cholesterol levels."

Most recently, the Academy of Nutrition and Dietetics (2016) have updated their position of vegetarian (and vegan diets) to further add, "Plant-based diets are more environmentally sustainable than diets rich in animal products because they use fewer natural resources and are associated with much less environmental damage." The organization still recognizes that vegan diets are healthy in all stages of life as well.

Along the same lines, Dieticians of Canada states, "A healthy vegan diet can meet all your nutrient needs at any stage of life including when you are pregnant, breastfeeding, or an older adult." While they do also emphasize planning to ensure vegans meet all their nutritional needs from food or supplements, they also state, "a healthy vegan diet has many health benefits including lower rates of obesity, heart disease, high blood pressure, high blood cholesterol, type 2 diabetes, and certain types of cancer."

The Association of UK Dieticians also states, "Well-planned vegetarian diets are appropriate for all stages of life and have many benefits." Lastly, once again, the Dieticians Association of Australia states that "with good planning, it is possible to obtain all the nutrients required for good health on a vegan diet."

Other dietetic and health organizations that have made statements in support of vegan diets include Mayo Clinic (2016), Harvard Medical School, the United States Department of Agriculture (2016), Heart and Stroke Foundation of Canada (2016), Australia's National Health & Medical Research Council (2013), National Health Services, UK (2016), and the British Nutrition Foundation (2016) to name a few.

I hope this brief summary serves as a reminder that yes, well-planned vegan diets are perfectly safe for our children. Next time someone questions you about the safety of vegan diets for children or yourself, hand them one of these slips to direct them to some of the dietetic associations that have come out in support of vegan diets.

Thank you for your interest in my child's vegan diet. Through a simple Google search, you will be able to find supportive statements about vegan diets from the Academy of Nutrition and Dietetics, the Association of UK Dieticians, the Dieticians Association of Australia, and the Dieticians of Canada. They have all stated that vegan diets are safe and healthful for all stages of life, including children.

Thank you for your interest in my child's vegan diet. Through a simple Google search, you will be able to find supportive statements about vegan diets from the Academy of Nutrition and Dietetics, the Association of UK Dieticians, the Dieticians Association of Australia, and the Dieticians of Canada. They have all stated that vegan diets are safe and healthful for all stages of life, including children.

Thank you for your interest in my child's vegan diet. Through a simple Google search, you will be able to find supportive statements about vegan diets from the Academy of Nutrition and Dietetics, the Association of UK Dieticians, the Dieticians Association of Australia, and the Dieticians of Canada. They have all stated that vegan diets are safe and healthful for all stages of life, including children.

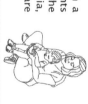

Thank you for your interest in my child's vegan diet. Through a simple Google search, you will be able to find supportive statements about vegan diets from the Academy of Nutrition and Dietetics, the Association of UK Dieticians, the Dieticians Association of Australia, and the Dieticians of Canada. They have all stated that vegan diets are safe and healthful for all stages of life, including children.

3

STAYING SKEPTICAL

I have found that many of my parenting worries since becoming a mother have centered on food. In my quest to feed my son, I have found other parents had many of the same concerns and fears that I did. What should he be eating month to month, how much, when is this or that safe to introduce, is this ingredient safe, what about formula, breastfeeding, vaccines, medication, etc.? These were the types of significant concerns I faced early on in raising a vegan child.

Every time I looked at a new concern posted on Facebook by a vegan parent, I started looking into it and found that many of these concerns were being made into issues by people that did not even have degrees or expertise to be giving the advice they were promoting within our community. The information has now become very much muddled with pseudoscience. Why is this of importance? Because raising healthy vegan children based on factual information should be one of our top priorities if we are going to break down the detrimental stereotypes that follow our movement. The idea that vegan lifestyles, including our diets, cannot be healthy has been furthered by stories of malnutrition, which although not representative of our movement and not an issue specific to children raised on plant-based diets, have carried onward. The spread of false information in our community has truly become a problem and has added to this idea that plant-based diets are not safe. Claims by individuals within our movement that go against established dietary knowledge and evidence-based nutrition safety guidelines have also added to this idea. This is why, with my science background, I hope to pass on the following tools to help you stay skeptical in the journey of raising happy and healthy vegan children. We already have support from dietetic associations around the world, we just need to stay vigilant and question some of the pseudoscientific claims that have infiltrated our community.

Facts, Myths, and Differences between Science and Pseudoscience:

Defining Science & Pseudoscience

In order for something to be published and accepted in science, something has to be researched, studied, and then peer reviewed. That means experimentation either confirms or rejects a hypothesis.

It is not biased and is only based on the results of that research through a specific scientific method.

In contrast, pseudoscience is made up of claims based on experiences by people, or people will make assumptions and link things without actually doing any research or even following the standardized scientific method vital to scientific research. It is important to note that anecdotal claims (testimonials or claims based on individual observations) are not evidence and make up a large part of pseudoscientific "evidence", which in itself is problematic.

Consensus in the Scientific Community

The large majority of scientists agree that climate change is happening (NASA 2017). Based on this scientific consensus and research, well-known organizations such as the UN have stated that to fight climate change, we should all adopt plant-based diets (UNEP 2010). Based on scientific research from groups such as the dietary organizations previously listed, veganism is supported as safe for all stages of life. If we are to believe scientists and available research on one issue because it is of benefit to us, why would we ignore well-established scientific consensus in others when it is the same scientific body that governs the same methods and reviews to establish safety guidelines? This is also important to consider on other topics, such as GMOs (AAAS 2012) and vaccines (WHO 2014).

Chemical Does Not Automatically Mean Toxic

Dihydrogen oxide is a pretty daunting sounding name for something, but it makes up the majority of our body, and we could not survive without it. The compound is also known as water. Water can kill you. If you drink it faster than what your kidneys can process, water becomes deadly. Even though it is "natural", water is also a chemical. In essence, everything has a "dose" or a limit before it becomes toxic. Complex sounding names do not mean that a chemical is bad for you. In some cases, scientists simply assign names based on that item's chemistry. Everything is chemical. We are all made from chemicals.

In addition, synthetic does not mean that something is toxic or less healthy. It means that the base chemicals needed to form it were used to make the same thing but in a lab with pretty much the same properties as the one found in nature. The difference is the one in nature comes "ready-made". Interestingly, synthetic versions can be easier for the body to absorb at times. So not only can synthetic compounds be safe, but they are sometimes more beneficial to humans. Let's take folic acid and folate as an example. I've seen time and time again statements that claim folate is better because it is natural, yet science has shown that folic acid is more bioavailable (easier for the body to absorb) but is basically the same as folate (FAO 2017 and Winkels et al. 2007).

I've seen one too many pseudoscientific blogs continue to claim that the natural version is better, but it's just not true. Some even go as far as to claim the scientific community is hiding secrets and keeping truths from you while trying to sell you their own supplements or meal plans. Next time you see someone writing blog posts featuring words like "all-natural", "toxic", "chemical-free", or "toxin-free", yet on the next page try to sell you their supplements or miracle cure, ask yourself if that person truly has your best interest in mind. Other key words that signal a big dollop of pseudoscience is coming are "cure-all", "toxic", "energy", "detox", and many more...

Manipulation & Misunderstanding of Studies

Misrepresentation and misunderstanding of scientific studies are quite common in pseudoscience. Why would something that has been widely studied and proven to be safe suddenly become toxic?

In cases such as carrageenan, it appears that whoever started the myth did not understand that the study on toxicity, which is continuously used as proof that carrageenan is unsafe, was carried out on degraded carrageenan, which is now called poligeenan. Poligeenan has nothing to do with the carrageenan that is widely used in toothpaste and ice creams. Carrageenan is safe (Cohen and Ito 2002), and the other (poligeenan) isn't used for human consumption at all. Carrageenan also has a safety rating of "no toxicological concern" from the FAO/WHO (JECFA 2014).

Another example is soy. This little bean has been a source of controversy in our diets – but why? The myth that soy is so unhealthy can be traced to the Weston A. Price Foundation, which makes unfounded claims about soy and promotes meat and raw milk instead (Wilson 2014). Those benefits may include a reduced risk of breast cancer (and reduced recurrence), reduced risk of fibroids, and even cancer reduction rates in men to name a few (Barnard 2011).

Even soy infant formula is safe. A study found that infants raised on cow milk based infant formula, soy infant formula, and breast milk, all develop normally (Andres et. al. 2012). The isoflavones (phytoestrogens) in soy infant formula have also been found to be safe and do not affect growth, development, or reproduction in humans (Russel and Jenks 2004). In addition, a larger scale study is set for publication in 2017 following the publication of this guide.

Carrageenan and soy are two food ingredients that have been extensively researched and found to be safe, yet have recently been demonized based on faulty information that has spread in our community - do you see a trend here?

Research Studies & Scientific Evidence

Unfortunately, there are such things as predatory research journals that publish articles and studies not based on proper scientific methodology. These are not scientifically accurate nor considered ethical in science. I believe this is where much confusion comes from about the legitimacy of scientific research and methodology when those who are untrained in science attempt research "studies" for themselves. Science speak is also never in absolutes, which can be confusing when reading scientific papers and in determining the conclusion of a study.

More importantly is recognizing that, in science, not all evidence is equal. For example, case studies and surveys are not definitive consensuses on a topic, and neither are single studies. The highest available scientific evidence is meta-analytical studies (or systematic reviews). These types of reviews are based on all the available peer-reviewed studies that have been done on a topic of good quality (well-established hypothesis and methodology).

To illustrate the levels of evidence, keep this illustration in mind:

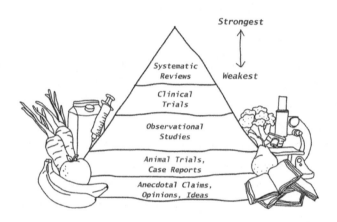

Bias in Pseudoscience

Cherry-picking data is another common problem I've found on blogs claiming perfectly safe things are suddenly unsafe. Many times, these blogs will quote a single study that isn't a real scientific study at all, or they will use research that claims the opposite of what they claim (that is it safe). Many times they will take a sentence and apply it to another context to support their cherry-picking data. This tactic is commonly employed on pseudoscience blogs claiming that certain things are suddenly unsafe to use or consume.

Experts Versus Unqualified Personas

People without expertise writing or making statements about things they are not actually qualified in is a common occurrence in popular pseudoscience blogs. I was in discussion with another parent when they sent me a link to a known unreliable news site article as their sole source of evidence for a claim. When I looked up the author of the article, I found that not only were they not an expert in the topic they were making unfounded medical claims about, but their actual profession was running an online travel site. Even worse, the "news site" periodically publishes anti-vegan articles based on pseudoscientific claims. I can't emphasize enough how important it is to look up the authors of articles that claim the opposite of what our society has deemed safe, even if they claim to be doctors. Researching news sources and blogs on their accuracy and legitimacy has become imperative.

Titles & A Lack of Evidence

There are also certain people that add "Dr." to their name or that do have a Ph.D. but make statements that do not follow science-based evidence. Again, if someone is suddenly going against the general consensus of the medical community and the scientific community, I've started to question what their intention may be.

In Summary...

I am a vegan, first and foremost, because I believe it is unethical and wrong to abuse and slaughter non-human animals when there are alternatives available. Obviously, as the definition of veganism states, we can only do this with things we have control over and are practical in our very non-vegan world. As a parent, we want to do the best we can but also need to recognize that science and the medical community are valuable resources that can help us continue to further our cause and help us raise healthy and vibrant ethical little vegans. Many of these same bodies have already written in support of vegan diets (The Academy of Nutrition and Dietetics, for example). Just because we reject something society does with our lifestyle (non-human exploitation), it does not mean we need to reject every other aspect of society.

4

SKEPTICAL VEGAN PARENT CHECKLIST

Here are some key notes on how to remain skeptical when you are reading through blogs and other sites and are not sure if they are reliable. If you find yourself doubting a claim, check this list and see how it measures up.

• Is the person trying to sell you something? Do they claim it is all-natural, toxic, chemical-free, detox-related, and/or a cure? Do they then link to their own supplements and products or books?

• Do a search about the scientific consensus on the topic. Include keywords, such as "evidence-based medicine", "evidence-based science", "science-based medicine", "pseudoscience", "hoax", "myth", "debunk", and "skeptic" in the search, for example.

• What evidence is being given to support the claims? Are they providing you with links to more of their own articles? Do their links lead to the front pages of their listed source and not a specific paper? Are they basing their "proof" on testimonials or personal experiences (this is called anecdotal evidence and is not proof of anything)?

• If you are provided with what appears to be a scientific paper, who are the authors? Research the authors to determine if they truly are experts in the field in which they are making claims. What is their trained expertise, if any? Please note that pub med links do not automatically mean they are from legit sources. Pub med is a search engine that lists citations for journals and books. However, there are journals that are not reputable and made up by non-experts.

• If it is a legitimate scientific paper, can you be certain the study in question actually has to do with the claim they are making? I see this often. A blog will misquote a study or use the results to apply it to a claim, but the study has nothing to do with the connection they are trying to make.

• Scientific articles are peer reviewed by anonymous experts in the same subject area of the article. Research the article and authors, but also research the journal. Has it been widely referenced by well-known organizations or universities?

• If it is a legit paper/study, you could also just write to the scientist listed as the main contact on the paper for clarification. I've done this before in my own research. It may sound intimidating, but I've never met a scientist that did not like to discuss their work.

• You can also look for systematic reviews that have been published on the subject. This means they will have looked at all the available research that has been done to determine whether something is safe, for example.

• Free can mean pseudoscience as much as someone trying to sell you something, so again, search the author and blog. Who is behind it? Are they are a biased organization or media, for example?

• Instead, look at what organizations, such as the WHO, FAO, and their joint committees have to say on the matter, especially if it is food related. A rating of "ADI not specified" by the JECFA and WHO means there is no toxicological concern (this is the case for MSG and carrageenan, for example).

• If you are truly at a loss, there are vegan science/skeptic blogs that you can refer to in your quest to find the truth behind a claim; they may have looked into the topic already and may be able to provide you with resources on it.

• You can also find science-minded vegan groups that are ready to discuss a variety of topics and help provide you with resources, but again, stay skeptical and use critical thinking when in any discussion. Always check the sources. Never be afraid to ask for peer-reviewed evidence.

5

FEEDING INFANTS & WEANING

The American Academy of Pediatricians supports exclusive breastfeeding or formula feeding until about 6 months of age – the stage when food should be introduced (AAP 2017). The Academy of Nutrition and Dietetics (AND) and WHO advise the same. In other countries, food introduction is acceptable from 4 months but no later than 6 months, as in the US.

Specific to vegans and their babies, the AND states, "breast milk of vegetarian women is similar in composition to that of nonvegetarians and is nutritionally adequate. Commercial infant formulas should be used if infants are not breastfed or are weaned before 1 year of age." The updated 2016 position statement states the same and adds, "complementary foods should be rich in energy, protein, iron, and zinc, and may include hummus, tofu, well-cooked legumes, and mashed avocado."

Because breast milk is low in iron, the AAP recommends iron supplements for breastfed infants beginning at 4 months until iron-rich foods are introduced (Messina 2017).

When weaning, the AND recommends "solid foods should be introduced in the same progression as for nonvegetarian infants." Meats can be replaced with things like mashed or pureed tofu and legumes. Soy yogurt and other mashed or pureed plant-based foods can easily replace traditional nonvegan ones. The Academy further encourages that between 7 to 10 months, bite-sized foods be introduced, including things like cubed tofu and soy cheese, for example. In addition, "foods that are rich in energy and nutrients such as legume spreads, tofu, and mashed avocado should be used when the infant is being weaned. Dietary fat should not be restricted in children younger than 2 years."

As for milk, "full-fat, fortified soy milk can be used as a primary beverage starting at age 1 year or older for a child who is growing normally and eating a variety of foods."

My son's eating journey...

Based on my own literature review from various vegan RDs and medical sources, this is what I fed my son, and how I will be feeding my youngest:

0 to 5 months – Breastmilk or Formula only

5 to 6 months – I started with baby cereal at night and

then added 1-2 teaspoons of fruit or vegetable purée at lunch time to get my son used to different flavors, breastmilk or formula for all other meals. It is recommended that iron-fortified infant cereal be a first food (Messina 2017).

6 months to 8 months – Breastmilk or formula upon waking, baby cereal and milk for breakfast, baby puree for lunch, which included vegetable puree mixed with chickpea or kidney bean puree, baby cereal and milk for dinner, milk before bed time. I introduced finger foods, such as peas during this time as well. In between meals, I would give my son milk if he was hungry.

9 to 12 months – Breastmilk or formula upon waking, baby cereal for breakfast, lunch was rice, pasta, or quinoa, for example, with a high protein, such as beans and tofu, and a vegetable. Snack time was mini finger sized almond butter sandwiches or a small slice of green muffin topped with peanut butter, and a small portion of natural, fortified yogurt mixed with fruit puree and wheat germ, and fruit, dinner was similar to lunch but with the carbs, proteins, and vegetables swapped.

12 months+ - Similar to what I was feeding my son at 9-12 months but larger portions. I made sure to introduce new foods (fruit and vegetables, for example) with his meals every week.

One thing I never did was force him to eat something or

finish what he was eating. For things that he did not like initially, I continued to introduce repeatedly every so often until one day, he decided he liked them, usually. If he did not eat, I never swapped out his food for something else because I had read that babies and toddlers have naturally fluctuating levels of eating depending on body and teeth growth, feeling under the weather, and other unknown reasons.

My son also received vitamin D drops in his cereal each morning. Because he drank formula until two years old, I did not start adding a B12 supplement until he completely weaned himself. His bloodwork always came back with normal B12 levels.

6

FEEDING TODDLERS

The AND has stated that "frequent meals and snacks and the use of some refined foods (such as fortified breakfast cereals, breads, and pasta) and foods higher in unsaturated fats can help vegetarian [vegan] children meet energy and nutrient needs." The AND further reassures us that vegan children are able to meet or even exceed protein recommendations despite needing a higher intake of protein due to the differences in plant-based protein composition and digestibility. This should be of great reassurance to us parents and caretakers.

The most important nutrients to focus on when feeding small children are iron, zinc, vitamin B-12, calcium, and vitamin D. Although deficiencies are uncommon, parents should pay special attention to the amount of these nutrients that their children are getting and supplement or add them through fortified foods to their children's diets (AND 2016).

Vegan diets are not about limiting foods. One thing I've learned in my years as a vegan is that plant-based eating is about variety. The same is true when it comes to feeding vegan children.

Simple Meal Ideas

I'm fortunate that my 2-year-old has been a good eater from birth. It does make me a little proud when non-vegan moms comment how well he eats his fruit and veg. He loves vegetables, fruit, rice, pasta, avocado, hummus, beans, tofu, seitan, and pretty much all other plant-based foods. He starts every morning with a bowl of warm cereal mixed with flax seeds, wheat germ, and a teaspoon of almond butter. He has two snack times per day and the usual lunch and dinner in which I swap out his high proteins, carbs, and veg for variety. His favorite foods right now are broccoli, avocado, cashew nuts, and fortified soy yogurt mixed with fruit. Of course, he very much enjoys little treats every occasionally, like chocolate sorbet, as any child would. He's a funny one in that he really enjoys spicy Thai food and spiced Ethiopian lentils dishes. Well-fed, my son is happy, healthy, has a huge curiosity for life, and hopefully, on his way to making the world a bit better.

The following is a simple guide of what I feed my toddler. It is meant to show you how simple it can be to follow a vegan diet without having to depend on complicated recipes or spend our very limited time over a stove.

At the end, I am including a chart for you to write down foods that you and your family enjoy that you can use to pick and choose from when planning your child's lunch and dinner.

Portions will depend on your child's age and how much your child eats. For example, The Vegetarian Resource Group's (2017) guide to feeding vegan toddlers and preschooler states that a child between 1 to 3 years old should have 6 or more servings of grains (breads, cereals, pasta, etc.), 2 or more servings of nuts, seeds, and legumes (tofu, tempeh, beans, other meat analogues, etc.), 3 servings of fortified soy milk/infant formula/breastmilk, 2 or more servings of vegetables, 3 or more servings of fruit, and 4 or more servings of fat (margarine or oil, such as flax or canola).

As for spices, I did not start adding anything to my son's food until he was about two years old. At that point, he became more adventurous and more willing to try new things that I offered him if he saw mom and dad eating it. Sometimes, I will give him what we are eating, and other times, I still leave his food un-spiced apart from some oil and nutritional yeast, for example. It really depends on your child and if they have demonstrated an interest in more natural flavors or more spices. It is good to remember that, our toddlers won't know the difference between foods that he hasn't yet had. So, something that we might find bland and unpalatable might become one of their favorite meals.

Breakfast

Breakfast is usually the same every morning, except on weekends, we might make pancakes or tofu scramble, which he loves. My son has eaten warm cereal since he was an infant, and it was always a reliable source of iron for him. Initially, I would mix formula in the cereal, but now, I use whole fat fortified soy milk. Each morning he gets a bowl of mixed Weetabix (It's vegan!), baby cereal, almond butter, soy milk, vitamin D drops, and chia seeds or flax seeds mixed in. Adding wheat germ is also an option if you don't want to use the baby cereal, as it is also high in nutrients. I started feeding him this cereal around 1.5 years old. Before that, his warm breakfast cereal was a simpler mix of whole grain baby cereal mixed with corn or rice baby cereal. There are dozens of types of baby cereals available with different types of grains. Most are vegan unless they have milk added to them. They also usually have very simple ingredients but are very high in nutrients, such as iron.

Check page 35 for our warm cereal recipe. For a weekend alternative, oatmeal pancakes, see page 39.

Snacks

My son eats snacks twice per day. He's an early riser, which means he is ready for snack time at around 9:30am. Morning snack consists of at least:

1 x fresh fruit

1 x dried fruit, such as raisins or apricots

3-4 x small crackers

4-5 nuts, such as cashews, peanuts, almonds, etc.

2-3 pieces of granola bar snack (store bought)

After nap time, my son will usually have another snack time, which is typically made up of the following:

1 x fresh fruit

1 x small peanut butter or hummus sandwich or a green muffin (see recipe page 37) topped with peanut butter

1 x soy yogurt mixed with chia seeds

Lunch & Dinner

Meals for lunch and dinner tend to be quite similar. For each, my son's meal will consist of:

1 x carb

1 x high protein

1-2 x vegetable (green and non-green vegetables)

+ 1 slice of avocado if we have some for either lunch or dinner

I make sure to mix and match different carbs, high proteins, and vegetables at every meal for variety. As an extra, if I am making pasta, I will mix it with nutritional yeast and a few drops of omega rich oil, or I will mix in the oil with frozen shredded spinach. I tend to mix in different things for variety. For example, with rice, I will also mix in spinach or different types of beans. You can do the same with couscous, gnocchi, or any other carb.

The following chart will give you an idea of how my son's foods are mixed and matched:

Mix & Match: Lunch and Dinner Ideas

Complex Carbs	High Protein	Vegetable
PASTA	TOFU	SPINACH (COOKED/SHREDDED)
RICE	TEMPEH	ZUCCHINI
QUINOA	EDAMAME	CARROTS
COUSCOUS	SEITAN	CORN
POTATO (MASHED/BOILED)	CHICKPEAS	PEAS
FLOUR TORTILLA	HUMMUS	BROCCOLI
	BLACK BEANS	KALE (COOKED/SHREDDED)
	KIDNEY BEANS	GREEN BEANS
	PINTO BEANS	CAULIFLOWER
	LENTILS	EGGPLANT
	MEAT ALTERNATIVE	AVOCADO
		TOMATO

Remember: keep it simple!

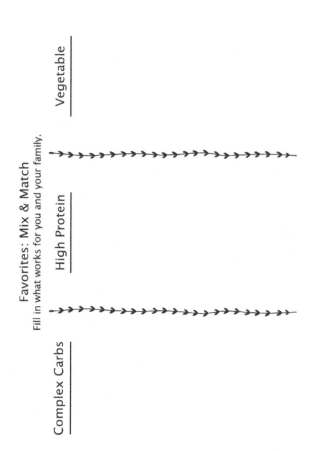

Favorites: Mix & Match
Fill in what works for you and your family.

Complex Carbs

High Protein

Vegetable

7

RECIPES

The purpose of this guide is not to serve as a cookbook, but instead, show you how uncomplicated it can be to feed children a vegan diet with simple and inexpensive foods. I'm only including these recipes because they are ones that my son has enjoyed very much. However, the possibilities for breakfasts and snacks are countless just by keeping it simple.

Breakfast Warm Cereal for Toddlers

Serves: 1 hungry toddler for breakfast!

Ingredients:

1 x bar of Weetabix

1 tsp ground flax seeds or chia seeds

Up to 3-4 scoops of baby cereal (your choice!)

1 large tsp almond butter

Fortified soy milk to wet the ingredients

Instructions:

Mix it all up into a creamy mix. Add soy milk as needed to get the texture your child prefers. Serve warm or room temp (depends on your child!).

Tip: Children's Vitamin D drops and B12 Spray or crushed B12 vitamin could be added and mixed well into the cereal as well. We currently spray B12 once a week into my son's breakfast cereal. It has a sweet taste, so he doesn't notice it's in his cereal (add AFTER warming up cereal instead of before).

Tip: You can make warm cereals out of many other ingredients and mixes that can be high in nutrition. For example, the Vegan Society (2017) suggests a warm cereal made from heated oats in fortified soy milk with added cooked dried apricots and pear pieces all blended together into a cream.

Green Muffins

Serves: 16 small to medium muffins

Ingredients:

2 cups all-purpose flour (other flours will work as well – your choice)

1 big glass (approx. 1/2 pint) 100% apple or pear purée (from baby food section)

2 tsp baking powder

½ tsp baking soda

1 tsp ground cinnamon or pumpkin spice

½ tsp salt

¼ cup vegetable oil

½ cup soy milk

6 ounces frozen shredded spinach

2 tsp vanilla extract

Instructions:

Preheat oven to 350°F.

Whisk together dry ingredients in a large bowl: flours, baking powder, baking soda, cinnamon (or pumpkin spice), and salt.

In a blender, place oil, almond milk, apple purée and defrosted spinach. Blend on high for about 30 seconds or until completely puréed. Add the vanilla; briefly blend to mix.

Pour puréed mixture into dry mixture and fold together until completely combined.

Fill muffin cups and bake 20 - 25 minutes or until a toothpick inserted into the center comes out clean.

TIP: These muffins will freeze and defrost well. I leave them overnight to defrost to have them ready in time for afternoon snack. I then top them with peanut butter or another nut butter that my son also enjoys. I only give my son half and save the other half for the next day that way I can also add fruits and other foods to his at the same time.

These muffins were also a big hit with parents during our early morning playdates.

Oatmeal Pancakes

Serves: This weekend treat full of goodness will serve about two adults and one toddler depending how large or small you make them.

Ingredients:

½ cup white all-purpose flour

½ cup oatmeal (extra fine)

1 tbsp baking powder

1 tsp vanilla extract

1/2 tsp salt

3 tbsp canola oil

¾ cup soy milk

½ cup sparkling water (for extra fluff)

3 tbsp agave or maple syrup

1 tsp cinnamon

Instructions:

Combine all ingredients with a whisk (don't over mix) and let soak 5 minutes. Note: The dough will be quite thick!

Lightly oil skillet (or use a bit of margarine) and cook until browned. Note: Be careful when turning pancakes as these aren't as firm initially.

8

TIPS & TRICKS

Batches of food

Many of the staples I feed my son, we eat as well. We mostly eat the same thing, but I will portion my son's food before I add spices or cook our meals in a specific way. This way, I can ensure I don't have to make a whole other meal, and we can still enjoy the flavors we like without worrying he won't enjoy them since my son sometimes prefers "naturally unflavored" food or minimal spices.

In addition, because we are so low on time and sometimes energy due to never getting a full night's sleep with a new baby, I will make dinner as usual, and if we have any leftovers, I will save them in mini portioned baby food containers and freeze them. This way, I always have something ready to feed my son should we get behind on our day. I started doing this when my son was still an infant.

Since infants younger than 10 months should not be fed canned beans, I would soak large batches of kidney beans and chickpeas, store them in mini freeze-friendly containers, and defrost them in the morning so it would be ready by meal time.

Split plates

I find split plates to be one of the most helpful feeding tools I have found. I use them to portion out my son's food and to keep track of different types of food he should be getting at each meal time, including snack time. I use standard 3 division ones, but I also have a 4 division plate for days that I add extra things, such as avocado slices.

Shape cutters

For an afternoon snack, I will make my son mini nut butter sandwiches cut into different shapes when he seems to be getting a little picky with his food, which happens every once in a while. It keeps him interested, and he even gets excited about snack time when he sees a little train shaped peanut butter sandwich or a dinosaur shaped one. I also have little molds for rice and mini cutters for vegan cheese and "meat" slices.

Supplements, Smoothies, and Frozen Foods?

Supplements

Vegan children can get adequate vitamin B12 if they're eating at least two servings per day of B12-fortified foods. If they are not eating foods fortified with vitamin B12, then a twice-weekly supplement providing 375 micrograms of vitamin B12 (in the form of cyanocobalamin) is necessary. For children who won't swallow pills, options are to use a B12 spray or to grind supplements into soy yogurt or other foods (Messina 2017).

Unless they have adequate sun exposure, vegan kids require daily supplements of vitamin D as well. Talk to your health care provider about this (Messina 2017).

Smoothies

We also don't do green smoothies. They may be a great option for those with picky eaters since you can pack them full of nutritious foods, but my son eats balanced enough that we don't really drink them. As for smoothies in general, dieticians have warned that although greens are part of the mix, many times, the recipes end up having very high amounts of sugar, which is not actually healthy.

Therefore, it is important, if you are making smoothies for your child (or yourself), to ensure a right balance of the types of foods being added into the mix with an emphasis on vegetables over fruit. Portion size is also important, as a common mistake with smoothies is adding much more food than one would normally eat in a single meal. However, most importantly, it is best not to depend on smoothies instead of whole fruits and vegetables.

Frozen vegetables, freezing foods

Independent studies have confirmed that frozen fruits and vegetables are as nutritious as fresh foods. At times, frozen foods may actually be higher in nutrients because of the continual nutrient degradation that occurs if fresh foods are not used right after they are picked (Barrett 2007). The studies found that frozen fruit and vegetables contain higher amounts of vitamin C, polyphenols, beta-carotene, as well as other vitamins and anti-oxidants, for example (Bonwick & Birch 2013).

Dr. Diane M. Barrett (2007), a fruit and vegetable products specialist at the University of California, Davis's Food Science and Technology department, states that, "a good diet should include a variety of fruits and vegetables, whether they are fresh, frozen, canned, dried, or otherwise preserved."

Therefore, a mix of fresh and frozen is perfectly acceptable in feeding our families. It can also be cost effective during toddler feeding stages where they eat small portions or show preferences for specific foods. Therefore, frozen foods could also help families cut down on food waste and save money. Studies have even found that canned foods also preserve certain nutrients in foods (Rickman et al. 2007), so we should also feel confident in using a mixture of fresh, frozen, and canned foods when needed.

Staying Strong

My son has discovered free will. We are at the "no!" stage – some, I admit, I struggle not to giggle at because he looks so darn cute speaking up for himself. However, with his never ending testing comes times where I have to remind myself to stay strong and not give in. This is especially true during meal times. By now, my son has food preferences, and although he is a good eater, he does try to test and see if I will give in and let him have raisins instead of finishing his lunch. I read a while back that toddlers will not let themselves go hungry, and they will eat as much as they need. My child nurse, which is provided free of charge by a parental organization in Switzerland to monitor babies' development in between doctor appointments, further echoed this same statement. I decided to give it a go and not worry if my son seemed to be acting picky because he wanted another type of food than the one I had made him. Guess what? Staying strong and repeatedly letting my son know that the meal I have made is what is available to eat for that meal tends to work. Sure, he tests and asks for a banana or more avocado instead of finishing his meal or even touching it, but eventually (maybe 10-30 minutes later), he eats his food without a problem. Often, he proudly announces he has eaten it all and makes a point to show me with a smile. I think we can be confident it is just another stage in toddler world.

9

F.A.Q. ABOUT FEEDING VEGAN KIDS

Do I really need to introduce food after 6 months?

The WHO and UNICEF recommend the "introduction of nutritionally adequate and safe complementary (solid) foods at 6 months together with continued breastfeeding up to 2 years of age or beyond." After 6 months of age, breast milk and formula are not nutritionally complete to provide adequate nutrition to growing infants. Therefore, it is important that parents do begin to introduce solids by 6 months of age (WHO 2016).

What is the best plant milk to give my toddler?

The most nutritionally adequate plant milk for growing toddlers is fortified full-fat soy milk. All other plant based milks are too low in proteins and energy to use as a replacement milk (Mangels 2017). However, plant milks should never be used as replacement milks during the first year of life. The ADA warns that "...soy milk, rice milk, and homemade formulas should not be used to replace breast milk or commercial infant formula" for children under a year old (ADA 2009).

Is soy safe?

Yes! There are already amazing resources by vegan doctors and dieticians that explain thoroughly, using scientific sources, that soy is safe to eat. Here are a few quotes about soy from well-known vegan MDs and RDs:

> *"Soy has been extensively researched – about 2,000 new studies on soy are released yearly...There is no evidence that this use has adverse consequences for health when soy is used in reasonable quantities as part of a healthful diet."* -**Brenda Davis, RD**

> *"Soy foods can play an important role in vegetarian diets. Tofu, tempeh, soymilk, and foods made from soy protein are good sources of a number of nutrients. These foods may also have key health benefits."* –**Ginny Messina, RD**

> **"Whole soy foods are safe and nutritious.** *I recommend incorporating them into a diet which contains a good variety of fresh fruits and*

vegetables, grains, and legumes." **–Holly Wilson, MD**

I encourage you to find these names in the references section and in detail, read through their past articles and research reviews on the safety of soy in child, adult, and elderly diets.

Is formula safe?

Yes! Andres et al. (2012) found that infant development of those raised on soy-based formula, cow milk based formula, and breast milk was normal. A study on soy infant formula by Strom et al. (2001) found that there were no changes in weight and height or effects on puberty or fertility associated with the consumption of soy isoflavones." The authors further stated that, at the time, this is the "largest controlled study evaluating the long-term effects of exposure to soy formula in infancy" and "no biological effects of infant soy exposure were detectable."

Is organic food better?

A systematic review, the highest form of scientific evidence because it looks at all available research on a single topic to reach a consensus on that topic, of the nutritional quality of organic food found that there is "no evidence of a difference in nutrient quality between organically and conventionally produced foodstuffs" (Dangour 2009)

Another systematic review of the health effects of organic produce found that "evidence is lacking for nutrition-related health effects that result from the consumption of organically produced foodstuffs (Dangour 2010).

As for pesticides, both organic and conventional produce are grown using pesticides. Organic being pesticides-free is a misconception in the same way that most of us, as vegans, are aware that organically raised animals have promoted a misconception among consumers of what "organic raised" means. However, if any, pesticide levels for both are not high enough for health concern. If any, simply washing fruit and vegetables, is enough to get rid of any residue.

Therefore, no, organic food is not better. There is no nutritional or health difference between organic and conventional food. It is completely safe to consume both organic and conventionally grown food. I've read too many parents proclaiming their guilt about not being able to afford to buy organic food. We already have many more things that make us feel guilty in parenting daily, and this should not be one of them.

Is an all raw food diet safe for my child?

The AND, which supports well-planned vegan diets for all stages of life has stated that "The safety of extremely restrictive diets such as fruitarian and raw foods diets has not been studied in children. These diets can be very low in energy, protein, some vitamins, and some minerals and cannot be recommended for infants and children (ADA 2009)."

Is jarred baby food safe and nutritious?

If you choose to incorporate jarred baby food into your child's diet, you can be certain that the food is safe and regulated. The preservative usually used is Vitamin C (ascorbic acid), and other ingredients are pureed whole fruits or vegetables. Cleveland Clinic (2017) also notes that "it is recommended to avoid homemade spinach, beets, green beans, squash, and carrots since they contain nitrates, which can cause anemia (low blood count). However, commercially prepared versions have been tested for nitrate content. Fresh foods spoil faster than commercially prepackaged baby food." Therefore, jarred food does have its benefits, including the safe introduction of certain foods, such as carrot. This is another one of those parenting issues that we should not feel guilty about, especially if we need to use them for whatever reason. For my own kids, I have used a mixture of jarred and homemade purees. Jar food is especially handy for long road trips or flights.

Is juice necessary in my child's diet?

According to the American Academy of Pediatrics (2017), fruit juice has no nutritional benefit over whole fruit, which contains important fiber and other nutrients, for children over 6 months old. Regardless, juice should not be given to children under 6 months. Therefore, no, fruit juice is not a necessity in a child's diet and should be limited to avoid it replacing other sources of important nutrients.

Is vitamin D important to supplement?

Due to health and developmental risks associated with vitamin D deficiency, supplementation is recommended for babies and toddlers. Breastfed children are especially at risk for vitamin D deficiency and should be supplemented; however, formula fed children should also be supplemented from birth (Kulie et al. 2009). Full sun exposure is not recommended for infants; therefore, partial sun exposure is not enough to maintain levels of vitamin D (Casey, Slawson, and Neal 2010), particularly of children that live in areas with low or fluctuating sun availability. How much and until what age will depend on the country where you live, so it is a good idea to discuss this with your health professional if you have not done so already.

How do I give my child enough B12?

B12 is one of those vitamins that vegan parents need to keep an eye on for themselves, as well as their children. On her site, Ginny Messina (2017) explains that "the only nutrient that could be a unique issue for vegan infants is vitamin B12. But as long as a mom is supplementing appropriately, her breast milk will be adequate in B12." Messina adds that "Toddlers should get a small chewable B12 supplement providing around 10 micrograms of cyanocobalamin per day, and preschoolers/school-aged kids should get around 15 to 20 micrograms per day."

Are periods of picky eating normal?

Fluctuations of how much a child eats are completely normal. As I mentioned before, it can depend on many things such as teething and growth spurts. In addition, pickiness about specific foods is a very individual thing that will depend on your child (Mascola, Bryson, and Agras 2010). Interestingly, science has found that some people are born with more sensitive palates, which will determine what foods your children may or may not eat (Dewar 2017). My toddler is open to most foods, but at 6 months old, my second baby is already "picky" about the temperature of his milk and food. He will actually cry and reject his milk or food until it is the temperature that he prefers. This includes fruit purees, which he is not particularly impressed by. My toddler never cared about temperature one way or another. He will eat his cereal either warm or straight from the refrigerator without a care!

As a small child, I wasn't picky at all about my food. However, my husband was and still is. Texture seems to have always been a big issue for him, whereas it has never been for me. Whether this will be an issue with our second born, we will have to see. Interestingly, a study by van der Horst et al. (2016) confirmed results from previous studies, where "tactile sensitivity may play a role in food acceptance among picky eaters." While the study concluded, "on average food intake of picky eaters differs only slightly from non-picky eaters, which seems to reflect a behavior that can be considered part of normal development," it is still very much important to track a vegan child's diet to ensure all nutrient requirements are being met in the diet. Things to try to reduce picky eating can include increasing the amount of times a new food is offered to at least 6 or more times (Canton et al. 2014) and not allowing grazing of food during meal times (Canton et al. 2013). Of course, the topic of picky eaters can be much more complicated depending on the child, so discussing any food issues with a doctor or dietician is important if you need help with replacement foods or further tips on how to feed a picky eater.

How can I add essential fatty acids to my child's diet?

Two fatty acids called linoleic acid (LA) and alpha-linolenic acid (ALA) are essential nutrients and must come from the diet. Most diets automatically provide plenty of LA since it's found in a wide variety of foods. ALA, which is an omega-3 fat, is found in only a handful of plant foods. To meet needs, make sure your child has a small daily serving of walnuts, ground flaxseed, hemp seeds, chia seeds, or canola oil.

Other types of omega-3 fats, called DHA and EPA, are not found in vegan diets. These are the fats that are in fish oil supplements. Although our bodies can convert the essential fat ALA into these other omega-3 fats, the conversion process is inefficient. Therefore, some experts recommend DHA and EPA supplements. There are vegan versions of these supplements that are derived from microalgae (Messina 2017).

What are reliable sources of calcium?

Ginny Messina (2017), The Vegan RD, advises that fortified plant milk and lesser amounts of fortified fruit juice, such as orange juice, can help toddlers get the amount of calcium they need in addition to the amount they receive from their diet. Messina warns that "It's certainly possible to get that amount from foods that are naturally rich in calcium, but many children will need fortified foods to meet needs."

Can my child get deficiencies?

Deficiencies are not unique to vegan children; non-vegan children are also at risk of deficiencies. However, it is important to ensure sources of nutrients, such as vitamin D, B12, calcium, and iron, for example in your child's diet.

Should I have my child's blood levels checked?

Personally, I checked my son's B12 and iron levels to ensure adequate levels despite his good development. This is something to consider and of course, something to discuss with your health care professional. For me, checking his levels was extra assurance that I was meeting his nutrition goals. Regardless, iron levels are usually checked at 9 months of age by health care providers.

My child is smaller than other children, should I be worried?

As with I have seen with my two kids, growth is also a very individual thing, and it is tracked at each doctor's visit. For peace of mind, however, on this specific topic, the AND (2009) has stated that "some studies suggest that vegan children tend to be slightly smaller but within the normal ranges of the standards for weight and height." They add that "poor growth in children has primarily been seen in those on very restricted diets." Remember that variety is key and keeping track of important nutrients in vegan diets will help your child meets their nutritional needs to grow as they should.

10

EATING OUT

Eating out may or may not be complicated where you live. I realize that vegan options are available more and more as time goes by. My little town has a few places that are vegan-friendly; however, none were friendly for an infant learning to eat or a very young toddler that did not enjoy spices very much. These days, my toddler is more open to trying new foods, and because we never stopped eating out even when he was very little, he will enjoy Thai cuisine and even Ethiopian dishes. Finding food on the road is usually not very difficult if we either pre-plan our stop or choose an ethnic type restaurant for meal time. Veggie pizza and avocado sushi with a side of edamame are also a road trip favorite. I do always make sure to pack both morning and afternoon snacks if we plan to be gone all day. If we are staying overnight, I will also bring my son's breakfast cereal already mixed and ready to add soy milk in the morning.

For that trickier time when he was eating but not eating everything yet, if we wanted to go to a restaurant, I would either pack his mashed foods and later, I would take a sectioned container and fill it with things like steamed peas, chickpeas, pasta, and other easy finger foods. I would also offer my son bites of our food; however, he was usually happy just to eat his packed meal. If we were on an overnight road trip, we would choose to go to places where we would be able to ask the chef for similar things without any flavor added. I find most restaurants are happy to accommodate a young child's meal. Indian restaurants are one of the easiest to order whole, simple foods from. For example, I've never had any issue ordering plain steamed peas or chickpeas and a side of rice. As a precaution, I also always packed snacks and always carried (and still do!) small containers of nut butter with me – just in case.

With a little planning and with braving a few questions, it is possible to continue to eat out with very young vegan babies and toddlers.

11

MEETINGS, PLAYDATES, AND PARTIES

When my son was 4 months old, we made a big move to a new town. I had to start from scratch. Three years later, I still don't know any other vegans in the area, so all my son's playmates are not vegan. The good news is that most people have been accepting without much thought. There have even been moms that have made the effort of making vegan cookies when inviting us over, which is always a nice treat.

Even with being the only vegans in town, one of my favorite things to do is to host playdates and little baby and toddler parties. After moving to our new town, I started having as many playdates and holiday parties as I could to become a part of the community. The only awkward part was tackling what to do when inviting non-vegan families over. Out of kindness, most people always want to bring food with them; however, that food is usually not vegan. Because of that, I ensure that with each invitation, the person knows that food and beverages will be provided and not to bring anything along. Being clear about this, I think has lessened any awkward situations that may arise. Also, because the food is provided, if we have invited someone new, the person's reaction is more relaxed once they find out we are vegan than if they had brought non-vegan food and suddenly felt attacked by its rejection. When and how I disclose our veganism to new parents always differs, of course. Some already come knowing while others sometimes find out mid-playdate.

As for what foods to offer, instead of focusing solely on healthy foods, I tend to try to mimic things that non-vegans would eat. I see it as a way to show the parents that vegan alternatives exist for pretty much every animal-based food. The ages of the kids also help determine what to make. For example, during playdates for my 2.5-year-old, I would usually offer oatmeal raisin muffins in the morning time while in the afternoon, I might have chocolate chip cookies and fruit smoothie packs on offer. It's always good to have things like nuts and fruit for parents that do not want to give their children certain food treats. However, the food is made to impress both kids and parents! I always enjoy the questions that come when they can't believe we can make baked goods without animal products.

For parties, we usually host brunches. This way,

we can have a variety of foods – both breakfast and lunch oriented. Mornings tend to work quite well for every parent that we have met so far since our kids are usually up quite early and the time won't interfere with nap time. Types of foods that we make also tend to simulate non-vegan foods; however, we also try to keep things as simple as possible because, with two kids, time is precious. We also do this to show nonvegans that making vegan food is easy and something that can be done with items straight from the shops.

A sample menu might be something like what we did for my son's little birthday gathering when he turned two – a brunch with a variety of savory and sweet foods. Apart from a cake, the party's menu consisted of:

- mini pancakes topped with cherry sauce

- a variety of mini sandwiches filled with things like hummus, vegan ham and cheese, vegan cream cheese and tomato, and plain vegan mayo-cheese. I cut each sandwich into 4's and then into triangles for mini bites.

- fresh fruit

- chips and salsa

- a variety of breakfast muffins, such as vanilla-almond muffins

- coffee, tea for the adults and water for the kids.

These foods seem very simple to offer, but they give a sampling of typical nonvegan foods with locally sourced vegan versions that can taste just as good. I also find that offering mostly finger foods also helps cut down on plates and food waste.

12

MEETING YOUR OWN NUTRITIONAL NEEDS

Taking care of ourselves is just as important as the care and time we put in to take care of our kids. Something that I have found to be true is the mantra "happy parents, happy kids." I know parenting can be exhausting. I sometimes find there are not enough hours in my day and the night (in between getting up for night feedings) is way too short. I have found myself cutting corners when feeding myself – running out the door without breakfast because I got busy getting the kids ready, for example. This leaves me feeling lousy and lacking in energy the rest of the day. I finally acknowledged that I need to take care of my needs too, so I am making the extra effort to make sure I get some time for myself and keep track of my intake of fruit and veggies too.

Like with our kids' diets, our meals don't have to be overly complicated. I start my morning with a quickly poured bowl of unsweetened muesli (a type of granola type cereal made from oats with some dried berries), topped with chia seeds and a good portion of frozen fruit pieces (I swap these every few days to keep it new). I pour fortified soy milk on top of it all and leave it to soak for a few minutes while I finish tending to the kids. I usually make it while I prepare hot cereal for the kids, and I make a point to take at least 10 minutes for myself to sit and eat it. Another quick cereal idea is simply soaking two bars of Weetabix in fortified soy milk. I then mix in chia seeds, cranberries, and chopped almonds. These are just two ideas that work for me. There are countless of ways to get high nutrient breakfasts in, so of course, it will depend on your preferences. My body appreciates a heavier breakfast to start my day, so these types of cereals work for me. I tend to avoid things green smoothies because I don't digest them well. I also try to avoid bread because it's far too easy to fall into the bread trap (empty calories) when you are in a rush. That's not to say I don't enjoy a slice of bread with almond butter or hummus every occasionally.

For lunch and dinner, leftovers are always an easy go-to if you know you are pressed for time the next day. I will sometimes make bigger portions the night before purposefully. Salads made up of spinach, baby kale, or other dark leafy greens, topped with beans or chickpeas and your favorite toppings are also easy to make and helpful if you are in a rush. This is something I will do if time has run out and my oldest is suddenly hungry. Here's where those frozen meals for him would come in handy while I prep a salad for myself. If I am too tired in the evenings, a simple black bean soup or minestrone soup works great. I tend to stock on a variety of frozen vegetables to throw everything in and not have to spend too much prep time on one specific meal. These are just a few examples that work for me. My goal is to pack as many nutrient rich foods when I can. I have a rule that, if I am also hungry, when I give my son a snack, then I make myself the same nutritious snack (for example, fruit, nuts, etc.).

It's an excellent idea to find a few minutes to sit (easier said than done – I know!) and consider what types of foods you like and can make quick meals out of if you are in a rush and find yourself skipping meals or depending far too often on junk foods. I've been there!

The most important aspect of feeding ourselves is making sure we meet our own nutritional needs. As I mentioned previously, as with children's diets, variety is key when it comes to vegan diets. There are a few key nutrients to specifically keep in mind, though. Vegan dietitian Jack Norris (2013) explains, "You should make sure you have a reliable source of vitamin B12, calcium, iodine, vitamin A, and omega-3 fatty acids. For some people, vitamin D, zinc, and iron could also be issues. Rarely will protein be a problem unless someone doesn't eat legume products."

13

A FINAL NOTE

Repeat after me... *you are doing just fine*. Parenting is a joy, but it is also one of the most challenging things we may ever do (especially surviving the testing twos or threes!). Starting our children off with the best diets and eating habits is a gift, and as you have seen, it can be done safely, skeptically, and simply with accessible ingredients.

I hope you find support and comfort in this guide should you need it. I'm excited to see what our world will look like in a few years' time when our children have grown carrying with them as much kindness and healthfulness as every human and nonhuman animal deserves. Here's to our kids and a more just world for all.

14

CITED LITERATURE
&
SCIENTIFIC STUDIES

AAAS (2012) Labelling on Genetically Modified Foods:
https://www.aaas.org/sites/default/files/AAAS_GM_stat
ement.pdf

American Academy of Pediatricians (accessed 2017)
Weaning Your Baby:
https://www.healthychildren.org/English/ages-
stages/baby/breastfeeding/Pages/Weaning-Your-
Baby.aspx

American Academy of Pediatricians (accessed 2017)
Where We Stand: Fruit Juice:
https://www.healthychildren.org/English/healthy-
living/nutrition/Pages/Where-We-Stand-Fruit-Juice.aspx

Academy of Nutrition and Dietetics (2016) Position of
the Academy of Nutrition and Dietetics: Vegetarian

Diets: http://www.andjrnl.org/article/S2212-
2672(16)31192-3/pdf

American Dietetic Association (2009) Position of the
American Dietetic Association: Vegetarian Diets, Journal
of the American Dietetic Association, pgs. 1266-1282

Andres et. al. (2012) Developmental Status of 1-Year-Old
Infants Fed Breast Milk, Cow's Milk Formula, or Soy
Formula. Pediatrics. Vol 129 (6)

Association of UK Dieticians (2014) Food Fact Sheets,
Vegetarian Diets:
https://www.bda.uk.com/foodfacts/vegetarianfoodfacts.
pdf

Barnard (2011) Settling the Soy Controversy:
http://www.huffingtonpost.com/neal-barnard-
md/settling-the-soy-controve_b_453966.html

Barrett (2007) Maximizing the nutritional value of fruits
and vegetables. Food Technology 61(4):40-
44. http://www.fruitandvegetable.ucdavis.edu/files/197
179.pdf

Bonwick and Birch (2013) Antioxidants in Fresh and
Frozen Fruit and Vegetables: Impact Study of Varying
Storage Conditions. http://bfff.co.uk/wp-
content/uploads/2013/09/Leatherhead-Chester-

Antioxidant-Reports-2013.pdf

British Nutrition Foundation (accessed 2016)
https://www.nutrition.org.uk/publications/briefingpaper
s/vegetarian-nutrition

Canton et al. (2013) Repetition counts: repeated
exposure increases intake of a novel vegetable in UK pre-
school children compared to flavour–flavour and
flavour–nutrient learning. Brit J Nutri. Vol 109 (11): 2089-
2097

Canton et al. (2014) Learning to Eat Vegetables in Early
Life: The Role of Timing, Age, and Individual Eating Traits.
PLoS ONE 9(5): e97609

Casey C, Slawson D, and Neal L (2010) Vitamin D
supplementation in infants, children, and adolescents.
Am Fam Physician. Vol 81(6):745-8

Cleveland Clinic (accessed 2017) Feeding Your Baby:
http://my.clevelandclinic.org/childrens-hospital/health-
info/ages-stages/baby/hic-Feeding-Your-Baby

Cohen SM & Ito N (2002) A critical review of the
toxicological effects of carrageenan and processed
eucheuma seaweed on the gastrointestinal tract. Crit
Rev Toxicol. Vol 32(5):413-44.

Dangour (2009) Nutritional quality of organic foods: a systematic review. Am J Clin Nutr. 90(3):680-5

Dangour (2010) Nutrition-related health effects of organic foods: a systematic review. Am J Clin Nutr. 92(1):203-10

Davis, Brenda (2015) Is Soy Safe? http://www.brendadavisrd.com/is-soy-safe/

Dewar (accessed 2017) The Science of Picky Eaters: http://www.parentingscience.com/picky-eaters.html

Dieticians Association of Australia (accessed 2016) Vegan Diets: http://daa.asn.au/for-the-public/smart-eating-for-you/nutrition-a-z/vegan-diets/

Dietitians of Canada (2014) Eating Guidelines for Vegans: http://www.dietitians.ca/Your-Health/Nutrition-A-Z/Vegetarian-Diets/Eating-Guidelines-for-Vegans.aspx

FAO (accessed 2017) Folate and folic acid: http://www.fao.org/docrep/004/y2809e/y2809e0a.htm#bm10.5

Harvard Medical School (accessed 2016) http://www.health.harvard.edu/staying-healthy/becoming-a-vegetarian

Heart and Stroke Foundation of Canada (accessed 2016)

http://www.heartandstroke.ca/get-healthy/healthy-eating/specific-diets/for-vegetarians

JECFA (2014) Joint FAO/WHO Expert Committee on Food Additives, Seventy-ninth meeting, Geneva, Summary & Conclusions: http://www.fao.org/3/a-at861e.pdf

Kulie, et al. (2009) Vitamin D: An evidence-based review. J Am Board Fam Med. Vol 22(6): 698-706

Mangels, R (accessed 2017) Feeding Vegan Kids: http://www.vrg.org/nutshell/kids.php

Mascola, Bryson, & Agras (2010) Picky eating during childhood: A longitudinal study to age 11-years. Eat Behav. Vol 11(4): 253–257

Mayo Clinic (accessed 2016): http://www.mayoclinic.org/healthy-lifestyle/nutrition-and-healthy-eating/in-depth/art-20046446

Messina, V (accessed 2017) A Healthy Start for Vegan Children: http://www.theveganrd.com/2012/11/a-healthy-start-for-vegan-children.html

Messina, V (2017) Personal Communication

Messina, V (2017) Safety of Soy Foods: http://vegetariannutrition.net/docs/Soy-Safety.pdf

NASA (accessed 2017) Scientific Consensus: Earth's climate is warming: http://climate.nasa.gov/scientific-consensus

National Health & Medical Research Council (2013), accessed 2016 https://www.eatforhealth.gov.au/sites/default/files/files/the_guidelines/n55_australian_dietary_guidelines.pdf

National Health Services (accessed 2016) http://www.nhs.uk/Livewell/Vegetarianhealth/Pages/Vegandiets.aspx

Norris, Jack (2013) Vegan Dieticians For Life, Vegan Views: http://www.veganviews.org.uk/veganviews127.pdf

Rickman et. al. (2007) http://ucce.ucdavis.edu/files/datastore/234-779.pdf

Strom et. al. (2001) Exposure to Soy-Based Formula in Infancy and Endocrinological and Reproductive Outcomes in Young Adulthood. JAMA. 286(7):807-814

UNEP (2010): Assessing the Environmental Impacts of Consumption and Production Report: http://www.unep.org/resourcepanel/Portals/24102/PDFs/PriorityProductsAndMaterials_Report.pdf

United States Department of Agriculture (accessed

2016) https://www.choosemyplate.gov/tips-vegetarians

Russel M and Jenks B (2004) Safety of Soy-Based Infant Formulas Containing Isoflavones: The Clinical Evidence. J. Nutr. Vol. 134(5):1220S-1224S

WHO (2014) Global Vaccine Safety: http://www.who.int/vaccine_safety/publications/aefi_su rveillance/en

WHO (2016) Infant & Young Child Feeding, http://who.int/mediacentre/factsheets/fs342/en/

Wilson (2014) A Vegan Doctor Addresses Soy Myths and Misinformation: http://freefromharm.org/health-nutrition/vegan-doctor-addresses-soy-myths-and-misinformation/

Winkels et. al. (2007) Bioavailability of food folates is 80% of that of folic acid. Am J Clin Nutr. 85(2):465-73

Van der Horst et al. (2016) Picky eating: Associations with child eating characteristics and food intake. Appetite. Vol 103 (1): 286–293

Vegan Society (accessed 2017) Vegan Babies and Children https://www.vegansociety. com/sites/default/files/Dietary_Guide_Vegan_Babies%2 BChildren.pdf

Vegetarian Resource Group (accessed 2017) Feeding Vegan Kids, http://www.vrg.org/nutshell/kids.php

JULIA FELIZ BRUECK

15

ABOUT THE AUTHOR

Julia Feliz Brueck is a mom of two and a vegan since 2008. Her education and professional background are in the fields of science and research, and she also holds two diplomas in art illustration.

Julia is also a published author and illustrator within magazines and books, including the first ever vegan-themed board book for babies and toddlers, *Libby Finds Vegan Sanctuary*.

Receive updates about Julia's upcoming work, books, events, and more at *www.juliafeliz.com* or on Facebook under *Julia Feliz Brueck*.

JULIA FELIZ BRUECK

"If I thought they expected it, they'd be less likely to get it," returned McPherson. "You can be jolly sure of that."

"What big teeth you have, grandmother," said Dave Yeoman. "The better to eat you with, my dear."

"Sloth," said Tom thoughtfully. "I wonder if I ever did preach on sloth. If I haven't, why haven't I?"

"Because you're too slothful yourself," said Dave. He reached for another doughnut from the thick crockery plate on the counter.

Tom ignored him. "We Americans are such activists—. Maybe sloth isn't our besetting sin. Maybe we need sermons about trying to do less rather than trying to do more."

"Maybe frenzied American activity is one kind of sloth," said George. "Maybe I'll put that into my outline."

"What else is going in?" asked Baptist Dave.

George smiled and stirred his coffee silently.

"You know better than to ask that," said Tom. "Ask him on Monday morning, if you can catch him, and by then he'll be ready to give you outline, introduction, précis, and conclusion."

"Okay, okay, foul ball way over left field," said Dave. "Want to remark on what started you on this slothful enterprise?"

"The Prayer Book, I guess," said George. " 'We have left undone those things which we ought to have done, And there is no health in us.' And I got to thinking: people come in to talk with clergymen all the time about the sins they've perpetrated, but how many ever ask for help because of their omission sins? Lust or temper or drinking can throw a man on the ropes until he knows he's down and everyone else knows he's down, but who ever comes around saying, 'Pastor, I can't live with my soul's laziness for another day?' "

"Well, Americans are always on the go; they really aren't so prone to laziness, are they?" Tom urged again.

"Aren't they?" asked George. He pushed back his chair too decisively for any answer to seem necessary.

After they had gone, Joe Bynum—the Joe of Joe's Diner— turned from the window where he had been watching Sarah Sellers in conversation with Rick Hartford for ten minutes. He got the Windex and cleaned away ten flyspecks. And then, in an unscheduled and unaccustomed episode, he washed the counter from end to end, using Ajax cleanser on the coffee stains.

Ray Kendrick

"Ray—"

"Um-m-m?"

"Ray—"

"Um-m-m?"

"Ray, listen to me!"

He put down the sport pages of the Keyesport *Evening Herald.* "Well?"

"Ray, you ought to write to your mother. It's three months if it's a day since you put your pen on paper. You know how she lives for your letters."

He turned back to the Cubs and the Cardinals.

"Ray, you aren't listening to me—"

His voice was muffled by the newsprint pages. "Maybe I'd better call her on Sunday."

"Ray, here's some stationery and here's your fountain pen. Right here. You could dash off two or three paragraphs, couldn't you?"

"Um."

The telephone shrilled. "Yes, he's here. Just a moment."

"Hello? Oh, Jake, sure, of course. At 8:30? Yeah, that's okay. No, I'm not doing anything. Be right over. Sure, Jake, that's okay. Any time."

He folded the *Evening Herald* and reached for his car keys. "Jake wants some help with his income tax files."

Tears brimmed against her eyelids. "You—you wouldn't like to write a short note to your mother before you go?"

"Oh, Martha, I wish you wouldn't keep on nagging at me. Why don't you write to her?"

"I—I did, I have, I will. But it's you she wants to hear from. You know that."

"Okay, okay, I'll telephone her one of these times. Look, don't wait up. You know how ol' Jake likes to talk when he gets going."

"Ray—"